# OtHer pEoPLe ISsueS

## Get Rid of Negativity
### *Self-Help Your Way Back to Happiness*

PATTIE THOMAS

authorHOUSE®

*AuthorHouse™*
*1663 Liberty Drive*
*Bloomington, IN 47403*
*www.authorhouse.com*
*Phone: 1-800-839-8640*

*First published by AuthorHouse 11/24/2009*

*ISBN: 978-1-4490-1819-1 (sc)*

*Printed in the United States of America*
*Bloomington, Indiana*

*This book is printed on acid-free paper.*

## LIVE...LOVE...LIFE...

This book is dedicated to "Most High" for my life's journeys to share wisdom and knowledge to people everywhere I go. I am blessed with my children, sister, and niece for their understanding and love for me to bear forth fruit of my spirit. Sean you made me walk the mile.

*With Love...*

To my special people:

Now is the time to place yourself first and this statement apply for men and women alike. This is a very basic need in life and a very important rule to acknowledge about oneself since you know what makes you happy in living, in love, and in life.

This book is for self-improvement and is not in regular form because we try to organize our lives in ways but destiny is pre-ordained in which we cannot control. All we can do is choose our thoughts and actions for a higher purpose in our lives that hopefully will benefit other people who enter or exit our world. Ultimately, we are here to find happiness and learn from our pains. It should not be the other way around. Your purpose is really all you have in life.

In addition, this guide is not written to read on and on about any topic but the goal is that if you can't use all of the information then use some of it and apply it to your daily life. The fact remains that life is a "very" precious gift from God and sometimes this fact is taken for granted for whatever reasons. Acknowledgement is the key to realize your gift and use it wisely while time is left for you. No one should become more powerful to take or remove you from being true and good to yourself or others in unselfish ways that feel humbling and worth something in life for you. I thank Bertha, Charlie, Beverly, and my family for all their encouragement.

# CONTENTS

# INTRODUCTION

I was inspired to write this book because of my life challenges of how do I relate to myself in a relationship with another person or people who display familiar behaviors and attitudes that were not conducive to my well being and how I was misunderstood. Being the victim was always in my mind and how I tried to explain my feelings and thoughts to individuals or family members only to not be understood or even given a chance for them to redeem themselves through self awareness and or mutual agreements and realize what I talked about to them.

Being quite honest, I was always the culprit of others who failed to realize that my method for living was not madness but a string of processes and techniques that are true in existence if all would apply the knowledge to their being. I saw where the loopholes existed and tried to express my reasoning to enhance better relationships with individuals who were reluctant to administer change in their lives. Again and again I tried to come to a compromise with no accord on my behalf and discovered the only compromise was with myself to stop allowing myself to be victimized and become the successor to my own reasoning which worked quite well and listened to the voices of first mind who resonated loud and clear to me. I found out that true happiness comes from within and I gave too much to other people who did not accept my way of logic or thinking that always kept me at odds with them for failure to see the light that shines so bright within us (me). Therefore, I decided that if it were to be then it had to be me so I made practice turn into perfect for myself and realized that these issues were other people and not mine. So why let it take precedence in my life anymore and found ways of really listening to my correct and first mind to self help myself and found out my experiments and discoveries worked very well for me and applied this knowledge to others that I have helped along the way. I feel more alive now, not being involved with issues from others anymore.

# Loving You

*This message means to place all people, places, and things in your life which surround you to give you pleasure feeling the joy of love...*

Our nature and we as humans can at times allow people who enter our lives to bring a pattern of discomfort to us this is an unnatural state in our lives because it did not exist before with us until the involvement of another person happened. The sad irony is that we make excuses for bad behavior which incorporates games, lies, broken promises, irresponsibility, etc. the list goes on and on from someone else. Well, the key to loving oneself is self-realization in seeing true colors that illuminate joy or the haze of despair. Readily, they do exist while seeing and feeling in addition to knowing what feels good and what is not is an important factor to know the truth. Am I in a love situation or toxic?

It has to be a scenario where progress blooms. You know what makes you feel good inside and warm all over and that's the love inside of you. Love is sharing, humorous, unconditional, caring, open, and truthful to reveal only the outer shell of love. Love can be in a different order for people like placing unconditional first but the common thread is how do YOU love YOURSELF? Take time out with yourself and know what pleases you for once in life to find out who you really are in the schematic of the universe. God has made you someone unique and distinctive and you must find this being again.

Stop giving so much of yourself to others who really don't appreciate your kindness. Tell you what... don't answer your cell phone--- better yet leave it in you car, the house, on vibrate or something just so you get your point well across to yourself. This exercise will detach you from being on a satellite string for a change with misusing the cell phone. Make others wonder about you while escaping their neediness because you always come to the rescue. Let their problems remain their problems. ESCAPE BABY!!! Let me make this clear--- get out of Dodge (Dodge City) because it is now your time to show yourself just how much you mean to moi (me). Quite simply, you have to learn to live for yourself again and make yourself happy. Yes, please use the five letter word HAPPY to you. Why? Because you love you and whatever is happening away from you it will still be waiting when you return so live, laugh, and love with yourself and you will become much happier as a person. Today is your day to start this journey and see what adventures that you will experience and remember one thing that it is all about love. Reality Check @#$%^*. What makes you tick? For example, do you like coffee cafés, films, boating, traveling or.... think about what are you missing that once made you feel good about it and you? Well find it! And Quick!!!

It makes no sense whatsoever to constantly place you on the backburner and sacrifice so much only to feel unappreciated and most times that is the case. It won't hurt others when you vacate yourself from being accessible and you will see how you are really needed less than you think. Make them take responsibility and make some decisions in life for themselves. A good breather creates distance which is therapeutic for stability with yourself and your focus will be much different to progress in matters that pertain to you. People become complacent when they have the same routine and that routine is tediously repeated and needs surgery to make it work differently. So the time is today and don't feel guilty about making the change or when you come home either because only change in yourself will set you free... memories are never ceased. Don't feel guilty about lovin' yourself or the choice that you made because at this moment it is all about you and no one else. So smile for a change and quit taking everything so seriously and relax, enjoy, mellow, chill, be cool, and rejuvenate please or you will self destruct and no one will actually really care. The worse thing to do is to allow you to become bitter and lose the joy of life and laughter. You only have one life to live so brush the dust off yourself and find love again for self. Kick the dust from your feet and keep moving in time and space because you are now in a place of passing through your trial or tribulation to a valley filled with joy and peace of mind in the land of milk and honey.

You can have a relationship or relationships with others and somewhere down the line you lose yourself and what is really important to you get pushed behind or maybe not even considered because your thoughts are always for others who you surround. Other people and their personalities can become draining for you and self is eventually lost and waiting to be found again. Some people have the personality of a vampire because of the negative dark side in them which indirectly directs focus on their harmful or damaging behavior and their conduct sucks you out of what you should be doing for yourself or another positive person. If this is the situation that you are in then make the switch for happiness whenever the need is there because it is okay and alright to do for you. When you don't feel like being bothered don't be bothered by people. You've been bothered long enough so why keep that fire burning? Just get the positive extinguisher and put out that pesky fire. How old is that fire? Come on now tell the truth. So you need to heed this message and beware of exactly what is going on with you.

Now since we have discussed and thought about loving yourself BELIEVE it takes practice and resistance because temptation is always present. Believe me it's the truth because as soon as you tell yourself today is your day then an interruption rears its ugly face, but remain steadfast and tell yourself, so what! Whatever! I'm still going to move forward with my plans today no matter what happens and I can't get weak and forget me again. Resist temptation and it shall flee even if you have to repeat this phrase to yourself over until it is embedded into your psyche. Let the situation take care of its own self and by any means remain positive and happy because love is not a chain around your neck; it is food for your soul. You know when you feel love or being loved because it is warm, happy, funny, exciting, and you feel unexplainable chills run inside of you. Love is amongst one of the greatest gifts that we have in life beside the essence of waking up to witness and praise God for another day in a right mind, health, and strength.

Until one knows the feeling of love one will never know how to love, love in unselfish thinking and most people thrive in a small realm of me, myself, and I thinking which decreases blessings for them. To love is to let go and move forward. Do your thing for a change. Have the utmost faith in God that you can do this thing that is placed before you because you are now walking in the part of your life which is your destiny and faith in yourself. Feel this path and move forward in it and don't stray. This will guarantee instant success and if it is practiced then you will see grave results and be able to help someone else who may face a negative person in their life. This may sound repetitious but really it's highly needed; re-enforcement is the key till you make yourself a habit that comes naturally and watch your world brighten up. Stop placing yourself out in the cold again, please.

# THE CHAPTER TWO

# Love

*Love is many things but to be in love is another...*

Love is about giving and sharing sprinkled with caring. You know this book could be ridden with stories of how examples relate to a topic but that's boring and the message is written within the words in this text so it is important for you to pick and choose them wisely to apply in your personal life. When exploring and finalizing love, one must first know and feel first hand exactly what love is? Remember the exact times when you felt love from someone in a situation and how you responded (emotionally, spiritually, physically, or mentally). When you recall those stimuli then savor the flavor because they are the guiding light to the rest of your life and how you allow people or relationships to approach or exist in your realm. Your realm is your life

7

which is very precious to you like whatever means the most in your existence. If you forget this sensation then you have allowed yourself to remain in the problem and sooner or later it will consume you whereas despair and depression will stagnate your being and you become a slave to ill behavior and can think it is the norm. So with all that said and done now is the time to make love last and nobody can control it but you.

So here's the challenge, if you love yourself but don't feel the love around you that you give to others. Remove yourself quickly for your own sanity! Oh by far, it's not selfish but it is a "self"-ish thing to do. You must take time away that others spend not appreciating you, nagging you, giving you problems--- transition is the key thought because the fact remain that you don't possess the ill behavior or problems; it's the toxic people who do. Basically, misery loves company so stop being miserable by accompanying misery from other people. Ask yourself, "Why have I allowed myself to linger in other people issues that are not mine when I have already given the needed answer that is not being used?" Do things that please you and fight the good fight of temptation to not involve yourself into the issues that you feel no love in it. Practice makes perfect. You need to surround yourself with people made of iron because iron sharpens iron. Good people stimulate and encourage growth in others by giving good counsel from having wisdom.

It is okay to tell excuses to others on your behalf in order to not let them bother you because this is a form of protection and self elevation   Okay so when you're on the cell phone and caller ID reveals "Le Misery Bad Conduct's" phone number--- oh well allow it to go to voicemail and retrieve it whenever because if it is really important then you'll get several subsequent calls. If not important it's already taken care of in voicemail. Listen to the message when you feel like listening but more than likely it's probably nothing. Whoa! You feel great now. Feel your own love and smile or kiss yourself on the hand. It is really okay and who is better off now than you. Furthermore, what you have begun is to unleash love from you to you. Good, your first time doing what you said you were going to do is to love yourself and make others try to see the light. Great! This can be your first time doing what you said you were going to do the right way and your way with better consequences. In turn, others have no choice but to see your luminosity or not but either way it goes it is not about the parasitic person anymore and remember it is about your love for "self" that takes precedence above all.

## THE CHAPTER THREE

# Issues

*Issue over here... issue over there these issues aren't going anywhere...*

Issues, issues, issues are another topic. You can get rich if you received a dollar from other people issues in which you are associated with. One thing about issues especially if they are not yours then don't be bothered. And then they become what? Powerless. You can change the subject, leave the room, refuse to answer, laugh, turn on the TV or radio, do anything positive for yourself so you don't have to listen and absorb someone else's issues, attitude, childishness, immaturity, and on and on. Look! You only have two issues and that is to remain on your target of self-realization and be true to self.

You need to remind yourself, "No, I was not concerned better yet bothered with that until you came into the picture so I must get it away from me." Matter of fact when the noxious person gets better I'll call then because my life doesn't involve that. This is not personal just business and especially my business that involves relieving issues that are not mine. So breaking away is the step forward for you and it is guaranteed that the issue will disappear. Oh how sweet it feels of victory. Rejoice and make merry noises to yourself. You deserve it because you'll even look better because feeling better is what's happening to you right now so don't stop practicing better habits.

Issues come in various forms and if you have to work around someone with issues then it is far better to remain professional and make as little communication as needed so it will not allow room for discontent or a loose tongue from you. Say hi and bye. With very little in between because this is a positive measure for you and you are in control of the situation. Leave them wondering. Bravo. Feel better Boo? Ironically, negative people have been in the damper of life so long that they thrive in idleness of human nature and can't quite possibly find out how to maintain healthy relationships. Negative people see being whishy-washy and changing from nice to obnoxious as a norm in a relationship and have a false misrepresentation that they really care about another person. This is a misnomer because in a fit relationship two people can compromise and advance in circumstances for the wheel of progression to exert contentment and fulfillment to all involved. It is better early on in a relationship to know exactly what you are and are not going to be bothered with from someone else. You must place a time limit on how long you will give them to grow or grow up and face the negativity issues face to face for once and all. If the fact remains that the growth is taking years then sorrowfully this has also taken years away from your life to find pleasure, peace, and happiness is not healthy for you.

The best way to deal with issues is to stop them before they get started and have a clear understanding with the negative person of what you absolutely will not tolerate. Early in the relationship this is a metric that can be utilized because now you are in the control seat of your life and have all rights and responsibilities of how far you will allow another to go against your well-being. Prolong periods of non-productiveness of depleting issues can wear and tear on your mind, body, and soul if you don't get a grip. So take the plunge and don't be afraid of what someone will think of you because at the end they can't do anything but think well of you and most of all you for yourself. He who laughs does not get the last laugh.

## THE CHAPTER FOUR

# Making a Decision

*It's time to call in the troops...*

First you have to stand up for what you believe in and your happiness moreover life comes first. It is called de-tach-" me"-nt. Me are the key letters in the word because you know your feeling of comfort, relaxation, or goodness that makes you feel superior and secure about yourself for a cure. Negative people and negative actions really do deserve to gain re-"act"-ion from you and the "act" is a decision. Many times you have made a decision about how you will solve an issue that another person brings into your world and many times you accept the same dried up apology and negative pattern from that individual while a promise to change is made but the habit only re-app-"ears". Yes, "ears" is the word. What? Ears you heard it. Now it's time to see that your decision has to be executed even though it may feel funny to you but only you can control yourself and create your wall and empire of happiness.

Do what you told yourself to do even if it means being alone for awhile, not going grocery shopping with the negative person or what ever first mind told you to do. Do it! All is fair for you to do what you feel is right for your salvation and sanity to keep your world in a brighter place this can be the only way. And by all means don't feel guilty about any of your actions because you have been on the forgiving end too many times and remember it was you who felt the jolt of negative energy that tried to surge your world. The parasitic person thinks it is a game now because of the pattern of negativity, apology then negativity again. You are the only one who can stop this trail of madness once and for all. It will take contemplation and will power plus some prayers for strength because this a step in the corrective direction that you have failed to execute and you are somewhat to blame for this issues as well. It should not have lasted as long as it did. Bottom line is someone is going to have to be the bigger person and say enough is too much and that person is you.

Please remember that in your world you love a certain way and certain things feel good to you that you feel good about yourself and you apply them everyday in your life. So feel good about your decision to go the other way and not feel guilty. Why feel guilty? It was not you who created the negative situation in the first place. So love yourself and move on to continue happiness in your life because you only have one life to live. Smile. Feel peace, love, goodness 'cause you're all those elements and much more.

Realization comes to know that your life must have elevation and the only one who controls that is you. You have the power to make things happen in your own way. You must know that you do have the final word and this is the essence to making a decision that later you'll find out work so well for you. By taking a stance and stop being the victim, you'll find a sense of release from negativity and it will disappear. Would you rather be in the house with a negative person or on the balcony having peace of mind? The key is listening and to your inner self and doing what is right for you. So when you hear that voice re-acting negatively to you use it for a positive to bring out the troops to protect your stability while doing your thing for self finally. It is time to get reacquainted with a better and more improved happier you. Remember a time in your life when you were most happy and how it felt. So now is your time to feel a happy feeling and an even bigger better happy feeling just for you. Look to yourself for happiness and make that decision and keep whatever it is that is good enough to make you happy.

# Talk To Yourself

*Me myself and I --- So you mad, huh…*

It's really OK to mentally or verbally talk to yourself. But the test comes in if you can listen to what you've said that you know to be correct and act upon it. Too many times, people have the answer already figured out and know the reasons behind the driving force to make a decision but allow insecurity to get in the way. Stop that this minute! It is played out and truly you know it is old. This book is a you help yourself book with strategies that will and can enhance your life from the same mistakes, misleading motions, or negative patterns that have plagued to you for who knows how long.

You are really your best friend and know exactly what you like and need so stop making yourself a second or third fiddler. Please! Take the lead! Would you? It's not that you're being selfish but you're being "self"-ish for change. Surprisingly, people, places, and things will generate a new consciousness in your mind for you and your mental state will increase as if you've deprive yourself long enough from rewarding you. Take the plunge into courage and listen to execute what your first mind has told you to perform. Believe in yourself and do what you need to do for yourself and others will follow your lead. Life is an open door. Have you ever spoken to a close friend about problem or circumstance and you finally developed a solution for resolution? Then this is the same scenario but a different player because you are left with yourself. Trust in you especially in times when no one else can help you or no one is around to talk to and in today's society there are far and few people who will listen attentively anyways.

It is better to take time in your thoughts then to make irrational decisions. We listened too much to others when your inner voice has all the wisdom you need to survive. You'll find in time a friend lies inside of you despite what others may say or do even better yet won't do. You have to be true to yourself because no other person can live your life for you only you can. When open dialog exists between you and your spiritual side you obtain clarity, peace, and movement in your livelihood. Take time for reflection in a quiet environment and meditate to clear your mind and seek the place where God exists within.

By talking with yourself, you can know how you see the problem? How you act in the problem? It has to come to pass for deliverance or you will stay complacent and dormant in the negativity that will take away your blessings from you. Closure is the key and your present and future are the rewards down the line for you to aspire and gain your senses back in line with your human nature. Take heed of these words because they hold the very spirit of truth for you in your life which is a daily gift. You should know that you are destined for higher flight to look around and have faith in you to remove all negative aspects out of your world to life's fulfillment.

# The Way of Others Is Not Yours

*Down the yellow brick road...*

Ideas circulate these days in rapid proportions with various mediums such as word of mouth, visuals, film, broadcast, or computer. The basic thought pattern is to sway thoughts to masses in support for people to believe in something or anything because maybe someone else has done it or it sounds good for the heck of it. There comes a time when you have to be steadfast in your standard and beliefs because the way of others can not take precedence over your ways for what you believe is right.

This thought process is not meant for being selfish but using rationality without judgment. It is sometimes best not to make comments on every issue but take time to reflect on the conversation and extract a positive solution to your actions without being offensive. The focus is to retain your integrity in a subtle manner where hopefully doing what is correct for you will get noticed by others but if not... then-oh well. Don't stop your impact-filled momentum that you are feeling this is your way. For a fact, you will know in your heart, mind, and soul that you have done what is right. Oh the benefit of joy and release; you know loving you for you and being comfortable to speak wisdom and life on a regular basis in conversation while giving these gifts back to others. Hopefully, others will acknowledge and receive from you and pass the torch on.

All you can do is speak peace and upliftment and the rest is left to the other individual. You cannot sway other people thoughts but you can truly roll off on others little by little till eventually they pay attention to either what you have done or said. Your life is special and unique which is meant only for you; uniqueness is different for everyone who seeks to find peace and joy in a society that thrives on misconduct and misconceptions as a norm for entertainment or reality. The fulfillment to plant a tree or flower or the need of water and sun to sustain life are basic elements; therefore, basic elements for you are reasons and enlightenment in one's thoughts and actions emanating from you and finally realizing how great you are in connection to the universe. Today, many people in general think because someone else has thought; seen because someone else has seen without rationalizing exactly what is really the truth. Their shallowness keeps them in bondage and constantly repeating the same horrible routine that do not produce any true or raw progress or enlightment in life. The question is what if thought or vision was not there? Now would their ways be different. Of course it would because the images that produce those outcomes would not exist which goes back to what was already said that most people reside in a box and believe most of what they hear without questioning it or using common sense which really is not common at times.

We live in a world were cloning oneself is the norm (i.e. plastic surgery, fashion, materialistic). But when you find yourself you see the true you really don't matter. What matters is being simple without the unnecessary added stress of a manmade life. Release yourself. There comes a time when you have to look at self deeply to see your own faults and how your faults are associated in afflicting others or others have faults that are combined with yours that afflict you. This is the time to be a leader and stop making the same mistakes and allowing another to help you make the same mistakes in a relationship. Don't be afraid because their ways are right now not your ways and it feels good to you to finally realize that you have been in prison for so long captured and living dead for many years. Be bold and stop yourself by going the opposite way even if you lose someone then this was the season for the loss because in all facets there is a season and a time for everything. A good biblical verse says, "Trust in the Lord with all thine heart and lean not to thine own understanding. Acknowledge him in all thy ways and he will direct thy paths." Everyone believes in something and if you sever a toxic relationship your approach is bringing forth good fruit (people) because now you know how to attract them.

# Selective Thought

*It is what it is and I see what it is...*

Have you ever been in a situation where you know the relationship is negative and one-sided more than anything? You make excuses about the other person's traits that are not appeasing to you but yet time after time you get hit in the head with falling stones saying where did that come from? Stop it! Please place that excuse in a bottle and sail it on the next voyage. Meaning, it is time for a better selection process in the relationship to begin. You can see the other person right now is incapable of change while maybe and will consciously undermine you. You do have the power to choose and say, "Hey, What am I gaining?" Is the conversation or relationship nourishing or have you found yourself growing and the insults towards you too? Say to yourself, "I'm to decide why are you here, why have I allowed myself to continue this pattern of negativity presented to me on a regular basis?" And why?

Your thoughts are revered and should be felt with appreciation and make sure others see this important fact also. Stop turning the other cheek to someone who verbally or mentally knocks you off balance who obviously needs you more than you need them at this point in the relationship. Use your thoughts to provoke yourself into something positive for you make a rule of thumb take to quietly extract yourself from whoever because you are busy doing pleasant things. Just plain busy. Short and simple tell them an excuse to remove your presence to be summoned to the throne of misery no more in life. Now you have released your selective thought of why I continue to roller skate with a broken wheel on each skate when it doesn't make sense? It makes not one minute bit of sense to continue this ride anymore. So take off the hideous bad habit of always being there for that negative person's needs and surround yourself with positive people who can use your thought process and gain the wonderful beauty of your true spirit that dwells inside of you. The value of selective thought is in shunning pessimism and be optimistic about yourself.

Routinely, over the years and habits have formed that may be somewhat in your thinking. You know your thoughts and how it makes you feel inside especially when things don't go as planned or when you're successful. Tenderly, if you don't bring something up (negative thoughts, people, or situation) then you won't think about it. And when you get those thought urges immediately catch yourself and say STOP because it is not worthy of your energy. Now the floodgate is open to meditate on something more positive or goal oriented. You will feel better and it takes practice to undo bad thought patterns. Time is your answer and making the right choice for your mind is essential. You know the mind is a terrible thing to waste.

# When You're Up
# Are You Down?

*Figure this one out and you won the million dollar question...*

Funny. Funny? Which one? Your choice. Life--- is sometimes a mystery. Life can be strange. Sometimes you have what it takes then again sometimes not. Now here's the scenario, when everything is going for you say people, places, things are exciting and you are excelling in your career or personal life. Isn't it magnificent that everyone thinks you're interesting; you are in high demand and people want to call or spend time with you? BONG! DING! DONG! It hits HARD and you're stressed or depressed and what is really needed is rest -- rest from life---rest from people and what ever. Ok so now your demand is lowered and all the so called friends stop calling or coming around because they don't have a need for you anymore because really when you think about it, YOU were the motivation for their thoughts and lives. They in actuality began to live through you. It can be a virtue to tell yourself that you made a positive dent in someone's life or dang I am sick and tired of people having no vision and using me for their mental stimulation. I'm not a psychiatrist. I'm not a career or personal life counselor. Now is your time to make the choice to allow yourself to remain getting used or to use yourself. Hhmn…a bowl of cereal and milk or bread in your coffee? You decide which one is better and by the way take the bowl of cereal and milk because it digests better.

The world loves a winner and hates losers and this fact remains to be accurate and awesome at the same time because we are creatures of prosperity. Unfortunately, the down side is that when things are going well for you some people become prosper junkies and zombies because of the materialistic views that are subconsciously in their minds. It is interesting to know how everything is going for you and how you had to take various steps to achieve your success for career or life but when the rug is wiped underneath you then the magic for them disappears and the attention is diverted to the next unsuspecting victim. These individuals have tunnel vision and are not really true friends because a friend is there for you no matter what and will encourage you to go on and move forwards against all obstacles whereas helping to create solutions for what ever is lacking in your life.

It is okay to take time away from everyone and reassess your values and how others are associated to you and what are they really offering you in the relationship. Are they fair weather friends or friends of the storm who can weather bad days with you? Be honest with yourself and find your way to a new beginning of discreetly weaning from fair weather friends and clinging to friends or family who are always there when you need them even when you don't. The time has come to free yourself from the agonizing thoughts of gloom. Surely you know people are around you because you are doing something they could never do or like to do but at the same time your best interest is not at hand. Peace of mind is worth more than a room filled with "take advantage of" individuals who surround you only for their selfish needs while looking for the next victim to latch hold to for as long as they can ride the person's success. When you break away you will at first feel a little awkward because this is a new beginning but as you continue towards freedom it will feel healthier and you've made a drastic recovery from people who do not have your best interest in mind or truly care about you.

# Pay to Complain

*I'm talking about you; you're talking about me...*

Don't get misguided by the title because in means it doesn't pay to complain to others. Really. Firsthand, the reason is stop complaining for one day and listen to observe other people who you talk to. Listening is the element of discovery because in their lives are constant complaints and really why should your circumstances matter to them anyhow? Notice when you are in their presence and you speak...observe that you really don't have the microphone on or speakers for them to really understand your misery about anything that you have said to them. So the best medicine is silence is golden and wow there's the breakthrough because no one is obviously in your woes to attentively listen anyhow. So now it's up to you to deal with it. Finding solutions and having faith is far better than to get slapped in your face without complaining when all you needed was someone who had the attention span above a circle to listen to you. Basic release. This is a phenomenal idea, feeling, or emotion that you will encounter and this is your possession because now you have another positive quantum leap of alleviating frustration as being misunderstood as well as not being heard literally from people who are in your close circle.

Release means freedom that was once directed to a bottomless pit of nowhere and now you're back on top because you now don't feel a need to express yourself to superficial or self- centered people anymore. You have found your Higher Power within yourself to depend on and listen to your every need. Knowing that God really cares about you and what matters in your life is always important including big and small circumstances. In society, people love to be around other happy people and misery loves company while some people dwell in lifelessness. Oh yes, you have it now you are at the point of creating new terminology of phrases for yourself to adhere to. Listen to you and wait on your solutions because a breakthrough is on the way. Rejoice in exploration of yourself and finding new strengths in life because you only have one life to live. Choice is the master. But one final message, it is OK to complain but you must realize it is the who you complain to and exactly what it is about finally realizing is it really worth to complain about or not.

The real thought here is why keep complaining about the same issue or someone when you really don't have to anymore. You are part of the problem because you have not figured out how to rectify the issue and may be out of wits at this point in curing this ill. Basically, it boils down to this and the answer is to not complain anymore but find a way to make you content and happy. You cannot change anyone but yourself so if it means that you have to sever a relationship then this may be a measure that you will have to take because the relationship is one sided and has no room for growth. Maybe this action will make the other person take a realistic look at the confusion that was added by them. Yes this is a drastic move but a calculated one because you have tried every possible solution that you could to resolve the problem and not one of them has passed the finish line to a compromise that is in permanent standing. It is simply time to move on or place the relationship in standby mode for a while for you to get yourself back in the mix of your fabulous life and get peace of mind which means everything in a healthy life, body, and soul.

You have to realize as long as you remain inconsistent you are babying the situation and the other person has no room to grow. It is the time now to let all adults be adults in maturity and thinking as well. A relationship is about two people getting together and communicating with each other while responding in a positive approach without a pattern of negativity of digression appearing continually.

# Best... Is it your best?

*At least I'm trying ...*

But really darling...how could you? Over and over again, you do it. Yes sweetie. You are guilty as eating ice cream and cookies while supposedly dieting. Caught. When will the elevator rise to the top floor or the light bulbs shine in your mind? You always give the best to those you love around you relentlessly and unconditionally of your love, but, you get misappropriations by the way of ungratefulness. But generally, you solemnly believe you are doing great feats and also sharing what you have to make someone else happy. Ok you have gone the extra mile of generosity only to get bombarded with the reality of they don't like it. What? Yes! After all of your thought processes, planning, and purchasing then without any gratefulness you see the face of— oh I really don't like that what ever it is when you know what was said in the first place to you that they wanted whatever it is. Well welcome to the feeling discomfort club AGAIN. Now the brain starts sending the neuron transmitters to receptors to keep your body balance and the balance is between your ears because you need it now to find relief. Silently you are upset. Your adrenal glands are excreting and you control yourself to remain calm because you feel fight or flight in your glands boiling. Later in your mind, the hypothalamus gland sends memory messages of previous occasions of best—Is it your best and are you on that narrow street again. It is OK to remember at this point because growth is waiting for you define yourself on this best matter for once and for all.

You have no other choice but to get your life in order for your own mental health. You should see by now what is healthy to others is not healthy for you. So stop the overdoing things and tell yourself NO to those best impulses that emerge when you want to do a nice thing out of the kindness of your heart. Suppress them. Tell yourself no not this time; I am not being selfish to others but "self"-ish to me for change my life. It is the only healthy thing to do it especially for mental stability for you and guaranteed to stop the counseling visits to the doctor.

The discovery is that you dealt with negative inhibitions that have plagued you maybe for years to rise above your feelings of stopping "the best syndrome." This will guarantee feeling better as time progresses. Now you have a sense of self-improvement because you don't waste your time trying to make unappreciative or ungrateful people happy anymore. Make yourself happy and the negativity will feed on someone else. Great! So now your best is your best for self. You will notice in time that things that you thought mattered so much for others don't anymore and you can openly express that and at first you will speak a foreign language because they will refuse to comprehend what you say. It will be guaranteed that as time progresses and you are dining, traveling, purchasing nice things for yourself – boy they will take a look at you and notice that you haven't bought anything for them lately. If they say something to you it is okay to mention that you have always been there for them and your gestures were not appreciated so you redirected your efforts to someone who you know will appreciate it. YOU! Next, bet on your last bottom dollar the sentiment has now registered and you can bet the next time that you do or buy something it will be appreciated by them.

Your best is now really your best and the greatest part about it is that it is finally on your terms. Sometimes in life we have to wake ourselves up to see the light we hold inside of one self.

# THE CHAPTER ELEVEN

# 2-4-1

*Did I miscount...*

This is really a matter of importance that must not get overlooked. Mental and physical health work hand in hand with each other and one is dependent on the other. How do you feel right now? Are you tired? Happy? Depressed? Stressed? Relaxed? Only you have the answer. Whatever the circumstance if it is a good one then you are ok and have conquered the 2-4-1 or if not then this area of your life must get worked on from the inside out. Your internal does affect your external. Although, you may try to hide your emotions it has to get released to find a new plateau for what makes you comfortable for well being. Visualize how you would really like to feel and how that certain feeling will alter your appearance into a new secure or relaxed person. This is an exercise in mental health to help garner a reflective state of mind. Now is the time to physically try new things out for you. The answer is that you shouldn't do anything strenuous or exerting and you may even need to consult your physician depending on what it is to make you feel superior.

Mental health is highly imperative because having elevated mental health improve your fitness routine. Your psychological health is part of your physical health even as a healthy sound mind is needed to produce healthy peaceful yet sound thoughts which are an important part of life. Don't think its taboo to say, "Maybe I need to speak with a counselor, therapist, or life coach." Now don't think wrong because there is in nothing unsafe to begin with a psychiatrist because maybe you need somebody who can shed some light to your situation by listening to you while not judging and will not make comments unnecessarily. In turn, you will feel much better about yourself and make decisions that you know you already knew that you needed to do but you never took that action to carry it out. Now you have a game plan with someone who is on the sideline to help and assist you in your endeavor to work out your new lifestyle plan of self realization or should we say self-actualization.

You will need to write down your action plan with your counselor and work that plan to the maximum since your livelihood and life is at stake. Who in their right mind wants to walk around being depressed, have anxiety, or even possibly think about suicide because you are surrounded by a negative environment which includes people? Typically there is nothing wrong with expert advice. Please don't feel like you're crazy because you sought help because you can't do it by yourself. You need to go into the bathroom and look at yourself in the mirror and say I love me---I make myself feel good. This is an imperative topic because depression or stress in the body can be related to a stroke, heart attack, or hormonal disorders.

Then on the other hand good mental health stimulates better body functions. Moreover, you feel more at ease with yourself, people, circumstances, and adversity which you can laugh at. Good mental health means you can build a better life style for yourself and people accept you as the pillar of confidence. Its shows in your conversation and the way you move through space and time because it is on your side and take one day at a glance for your life seeing that that is all that is given to us by God.

Exercise is a good too because you can go to the gym to blow off stress or even take a 30 minute brisk walk to keep you calm. You know exercise stimulates various brain chemicals that make you look and feel better especially when you do it regularly. It boasts your confidence and improves your self-esteem in addition to reducing feelings of depression and anxiety. Never forget to pamper yourself with a hot sauna or steam room session after exercising as a treat to you because of the serene effects that it produces for your mind, body, and spirit. You need to relax and let the other issues dissipate and meditate on self happiness of things you may need to accomplish or complete that have been on the back burner for some time. Relaxation and pampering yourself is a M-U-S-T, you cannot continue to live without it. Find what makes you peaceful.... Is it meditating, golfing, sailing, traveling or whatever keeps a tranquil mood alive and stimulating? Enjoying good company can be relaxing also. Do something different and invite a couple of friends over and have a cocktail party or go to lunch with someone. Remember the best things in life are free to seek out.

# THE CHAPTER TWELVE

# Own Happiness

*Go ahead with thy self...*

The key to life is to stop looking for others to justify your existence with the pursuit of happiness. Happiness comes from within your heart, mind, and soul. We look for love and understanding in wrong places; it is better to find out who you are and what you are made of to take hold onto whatever it is for dear life. Remember you only have one life to live so live to the fullest with everything and find companions who make you feel good about life and living. Quit allowing yourself to be around sorry, negative, and lifeless people or places. What a drain! Come on and be for real. Give yourself a break or you might have to take a vacation at a hospital with an extended stay suffering from depression because you are too emotionally involved with highly negative people. Too many times we allow unhappy people who never have anything good to say or know how to give compliments rain on our parade because we may fear controversy or disagreement. This is not the case anymore because you have to chip the ice and break the emotional negative bond with them to separate yourself and get your peace of mind back. It is extremely hard at first but DO IT! You are losing your life on a deadly rollercoaster ride that could end in tragedy.

Feel the sensation of happiness and make this point a target to always zero in on inside your mind to know how you feel so you can always make your own self happy. Don't look to others--- it is what you can do for you so don't blame others because they're not doing what you want or act in a certain way. Leave them alone and do your own thing. This is prime time to prove to yourself that you have control over your own destiny. You only allow people to have limitations with you because at this point it is not about them it's about you and only you. Feel this pleasure of luxury for once and for all please and then allow the sensation to become a habit for you. It takes practice and you can do it. Practice makes perfect and perfect you should be at keeping your life on track without the ordeal of always dealing with something or someone who causes chaos or conflict. Don't ever let anyone take this away from you because they didn't give it to you and darn sure should not be able to take it from you again. This is the key to a secret which is… too many times we look to others for self-satisfaction when satisfaction is "self" especially when you know you're a good person.

# Enough Is Enough

*That enough is enough and too much stinks...*

Look at the big picture of life--- what is more important to you? What is a big asset to anyone in the world with a stable mind? Now if you have a job that is filled with stress and you have tried time and time again to rectify problems with management and after months of expressing yourself while changes have not progressively been made this is the time to collect yourself and possibly move on. No more complaining about the situation and it is not self-demeaning to divert for better because you need to survive and pay bills. You also need to follow your heart within reason. You only have one life to live while you make your own decision other than end up in the hospital and have to pay the bill for years to come complaining. Find what is good you like and stick to those ideas until something courageous happens for you.

But believe what is it and think…would you like to pay the bill for stress and confusion from a direct impact from involuntary circumstances created by you? Or would you prefer to accumulate hospital bills from a source that was job related by people who don't value your service or human input? Well, truth be told if pray tell something should happen then it should happen because you couldn't control it but not from a second party. Feel better now because what you do for yourself is to be applauded and the action was done in good nature.

Our workforce is disastrous because of over work and under pay while this is where the line is toed. It is a shame that you have to stand up for yourself but in actuality it is something that must be done. Unavoidable. Now mind you that it can be done in a professional manner and listening to your inner self because self is communicating from a power within you.  Just slow down and breathe then pace yourself to hear and do as instructed and you will have power over your circumstances and never be afraid to moving to your next level. It waits for you to open that door.

# Fear

*But big bad wolf is only in sheep's clothing...*

The greatest fear is when you try not to do or a achieve something in life. People are strange creatures when you really observe them because most people are "yes people" always assimilating the status quoi. Never taking the plunge to be themselves and remain different. Now this leads into the fear of being thrown into the sea of outcasts because you can't disagree with the crowd. Are you afraid of being singled out? Called names secretly? Well so what! People will talk and gossip about anyone when you look at the big picture flowchart of life. Who cares! You should not because this is your best and is the precedence to use for all that matters. Point blank. You will find out when you stand for something you can no longer fall for anything.

It is a new habit to practice and see how differently people will respond to you. Analyze it. In life---, there is the ways of big mouth people talking nonsense and weak minded people joining in their lack of common sense. Just listen to some people for what is said and how they really act or treat others and you will see their bark is not as worse as their bite. You will really see that they are small minded and limited in their thinking and never finding the truth or goodness in life. Basically they are very boring people and have a lavish pretense for presentation of a life that is non existent and unhappy behind closed doors. So why bother yourself with wickedness or stupidity when you can love yourself and speak up when the time is right or not speaking can be profitable to you. Some people are so foolish and say idiotic statements in which warrants no response because it was just outright plain and simply dumb. Remember you have the utmost power to make a positive change and don't lose that essence because now you are the winner. You know you're the winner because you feel no regrets and no bond plus a new sense of freedom envelops you. Freedom to own your self-happiness which is a gift from our Higher Power and fear is only chaff blowing in the wind. There is no fear in fear it does not exist. What you used to be afraid of now you have conquered fear. Just go for it because time is passing faster and faster each year and you have no more time to waste.

# Mouthlessness or Mess

*Ole mouth can say anything...*

Time and time again have you told yourself to stop speaking to certain people or person because when you all converse into unconstructiveness on the others behalf? You say senseless you say stupid. Now let's take time out to examine dim-witted. It is OK to say these words and is mentioned in several passages in the Holy Bible. It can be bad when it's used to uncover reality for some. Let's say for the life in you that your goal is to be a kind and positive person. Do you live with someone or in a relationship with someone who possesses goodness and mischief? You experience a simple good moment turn instantly erratically into the horrid  disaster leading into hurt and pain again. Where does this come from?  S-T-O-P! Ask yourself.  Then do not go any further.

Learn the early warning signs and control yourself to protect your sanity. Well, you might say one last opinion and cease the conversation because you are taking control of the situation and not having your blood pressure rise anymore. At most through observation and diagnosis you have now discovered stupidity where you can control and you have the tools to leave the room, go walk around the block and comeback, or whatever. The key is to remember your self physically and mentally. Therefore, rolling in the mire with stupidity will only bring you closer to joining the club as an honorary member. So it is better not to respond to every conversational thought when you have observed the mentality of the negative person you're involved with. We are living in a day and age of self preservation. If you take time not speaking and listening more a new world will arise for you and what seems to matter at one time really doesn't have any relevance in your life. Mouthlessess was all you really needed to practice for this breakthrough in keeping the peace in your life. Wisdom says speak when it is really needed. By far some people love to hear themselves and often times it is about not saying something which is another subject in itself.

Mouthlessness means to train yourself not to get involved into downbeat conversations or actions and better yet don't allow yourself to react to it. This information may seem direct and some may even say I never use the "S" word but you have to get attention and using stupid in a positive manner should get the point across. Although, some people are stubborn and pretend nothing can penetrate but you share ingenuity by walking away from dim-witted will be left stupid all alone. In no response for the use of the "S" word as a lasting memory will be mind-boggling. Just say that was stupid then walk out when stupidy arrives and leave stupid standing there looking silly. At this point, you have your sanity back and peace comes since it is far better to have people call you for being mouthlessness then always talking or listening to complaints, problems, or arguing practically every time you are involved. You have to remain steadfast in your convictions and it may seem lonely at first while your need to talk may come but don't make the calls, visits, or start a conversation. Let people call and wonder about you soon you will see the light of welcome in your favor once more. It is better to be celebrated when you are missed then tolerated because of too much unbalanced involvement with folks who are not thinking like you.

# Room 4 Life

*Did the eviction notice come...*

How many times have you complained about the same issue over and over again? But you have complained so much that others get off the phone quickly when speaking to you or tell you they're tired of your complaining directly. Whatever the case you should be tired of hearing your own self complain and witnessed your happiness slowly sink down the drain. Realistically you've despised to get ready to do the very thing that discomforts you and now each day becomes a dreadful burden to make excuses as to why you still stay where you are.

People who are close to you have given you their reasons for your adaptation to misery and generously supplied their so called antidotes as to how they coped with an unhappy experience and the triumph. Wake up silly rabbit to see the light and notice that the majority of them have long since left their places of misery so actually what are they talking about? This has no relevance in your situation because in your world it is still discomfortable and your peace is still somewhat missing. So here's to life. You must make room for life again to live, laugh, and love yourself and other people who fit in your world. Everyone you meet is not suitable for your life and toxicity must be kept out completely. Now you can give yourself space to rest, relax, explore, or journey into another adventure of you. Life is so precious so why waste the gift that is given to you from our Higher Power. You are not meant to be unhappy and live your life unfilled while forgetting yourself in addition to living with heartache and headache in your blueprint of creation.

# Playing the Dozens & It's OK

*You need relief and security within...*

If others have relied on you but unfortunately it hasn't happened for you to get a turn yet. Your experiment for years has to be canceled because you're trying to find something that is not there. It is time for the dozens, meaning your time to fly moreover feel happiness to occur. You have always been around for others and their needs never messing up the relationship with lies, deceit, or corruption. Well the time has come for you and playing the dozens mean you won't be negative but you are on lockdown of your actions and emotions to safeguard self preservation. If someone you know doesn't deserve something is it OK to say no or you can't do it even though you know you can? You are not being deceitful only using your brain power because you don't always have to be there especially for other people who know better between right and wrong, When what you don't like happens over and over again and the same crap comes your way frequently when will you make the "AGAINS" stop?

At this point it is not the other person's fault it is yours because you are a number in this equation that don't add correctly. Release comes when you hear that inner voice telling a right thing to do is against your habitual grain. Do it. Relieve your self and if you say this is what I should or am going to do and then do it. Dang. You have nothing to lose and everything to gain in life, love, or happiness. When is your time for a mess up? Maybe never because this is not a your moral values and your character is more responsible and more mature so why allow irresponsiveness or stupidity constantly be a stumbling block for you? The question for you is why? Be quiet now. Being gullible is very demeaning. Yes you may have to say things that will make them gasp for air (but don't kill them) then you know you have made penetration then finally. The tough shell has been broken and this is the time for you to gain power in the relationship and maintain your new role.

You have tried different measures as well as you know who you deal with and what will have to work to get your message through. So being frank and theatrical can be an asset on your life's statement and somewhere somehow you should see a change some place. If not then the other person who you know will not change but remain in a stupid mode will have to make changes on your terms. Is the relationship really worth it? What are you really getting out of it on a constant positive level? Because you can do bad all by yourself. Remember you are self healing and not being there for ungrateful or insulting people will not alter you in being kind not one little bit. You do have the power to go to the opposite direction with your old destructive habits of always looking to help make a field goal for others. Well don't care anymore and put the ball back in your hands. Yes this sounds a bit cold but this is your cure all pill to swallow to get to know you again. The point is that people have to learn some things the hard way especially after you've rolled out the red carpet for them time after time. When will you get the red carpet service and if you don't then take yours back and give it to yourself for once to make it become your positive habit. One thing you can guarantee is that you will stay on top by changing you.

# Your Business It's Yours?

*My grandmother you have big ears…*

How many times have you told yourself that I should have kept quiet? Have you had your personal business thrown in your face or better yet gossiped about especially when you innocently confided in someone? We all have our war stories to tell but now is the time that enough is enough and too much stinks. Well really it does because like the phrase goes you talk too much you never shut up is true. In actuality, this knowledge implies that there is someone who dwells on mouth mail delivery telling everything about someone else's mishaps but never their own. They don't have any life because they live their lives through other people anguishes.

All you have to do is refrain from running your mouth and talking about your business. Close the trap door. Don't even think about it just close your mouth and not let it loose again that's dangerous. The running water mouth habit has to disband and is done caput meaning over. It's a curtain call. Some people lavish off injury and at the precise time will interject your hurt in a spiteful way towards you when all you done was have open conversation with them and now you know they can't handle not telling your personal affairs. That person acted so attentive the way you all spoke on a specific topic and it seemed as heaven had opened for you on that day because someone finally listened and understood. Only to find out later through general conversation from a third party about your circumstances or get it thrown back in your face. Your goal is that it takes practice for you to undo the bad habit that you placed yourself in by relying on the wrong person to keep your affairs private and understanding. Yes the emotional need that you have to connect to someone or people who you can bleed your heart to will arise time and time. But you have to know who you are talking to and what you can only talk about. Your breakthrough arrives when you speak and ultimately knowing that you are not revealing any of your personal information to people who don't appreciate your privacy. Most people talk someone else's business because they have a bad habit of gossiping and sometimes they may mean well but it is a hurting situation for you who is the butt of the conversation.

Then again, there are people who intentionally tell your affairs to make them seem like they are superior and always have the answer to every situation. Don't give them the pleasure of you being a yes person agreeing to everything said then your personal business is gossiped with a third party. You have to be yourself and not agree when you are correct if they persist in dominating the conversation just remove yourself completely or change the topic and eventually they will get the picture that you are not listening to any mess anymore. It's like who died and gave them authority?

# Expectations

*Not you again…*

When you look to others for your life circumstances you need to look again. Often time we look to others expecting something from them in return for something but you will find sometimes that what you expect never happens. It can be emotional but it can become rewarding to you because now you should be with the light. You can't change other people! Although this book is about you and you are the subject and you can only change yourself. Do not expect something from people and you won't get disappointed. We live in trying times now and social morals are at an all time low in the universe. People are becoming more and more self serving which is a downfall to mankind while the the more you do is less appreciated by them. You have to keep yourself sane and peaceful without much stress in your life. Expect the best from yourself because it is all about self-improvement learning what makes you tick or become ticked off. Expect the best of your self and others will see you clearly and at this moment you have rewarded yourself. You don't need identification or permission from others to feel self worthy.

You must expect the best from yourself and for yourself. Smile. Be happy. Crack jokes. It is your world that you build to your likeness to do what is necessary for you to succeed. Project positivity and really give it your all no matter what because better it is on the way expect means x-ing out leaning on others like in the past. Expect of yourself and see changes in your life and it will manifest right before your eyes to see a new self-personification of your pure life form. Try it and say, " I expect myself to do...................." You have to make it happen. No one else can do this for you but you only along with persistence is the key. The grip is broken because you are self serving even though you are around others but not emotionally. What you expect of yourself you can't blame no one for what happens to you. You don't feel disappointed anymore. Your world is bigger and better and a clearer picture exists. Practice makes perfect and you have to speak to yourself for encouragement to keep yourself on track to look inside for greatness and it will appear within your life by good thoughts and actions taking place. You have to do what you got to do.

# Feel the Fear Now

*Mama said knock you out...*

Have you made multiple concessions with someone you care about? Does the situation clear up permanently or for a period or yet never? Were you disappointed and the relationship rules broken? What did you say to yourself? Will you shrivel under pressure and not face the reality? Will you ignore the situation? Or...you can make the decision to move forward in and with your life. Having a will to fight the fear monster you learn to re-establish making good decisions from weak ones that kept you finding yourself going back into a hole again. Now is the time to make fear disappear by doing the unheard of which is to develop yourself in happiness to the utmost pleasure. Now it means you might have to lose something maybe take a loss; satisfaction comes in knowing that hey I don't have the monster hanging around me anymore. I've gone to a higher level and this mean that you have started doing things by yourself. Whoa! Sounds great because you enjoy what you do. The fear monster loves misery and misery loves company for these reasons it is time to let misery and the monster have each other. You have feared long enough and enough is enough and too much stinks. You got the power in your life to live to the fullest without any fear or walking on tippy toes big because of fear.

Fear has power when you allow it and when you figure out it is you who in actuality have the power. This is the rainbow to your storm with the purpose of an end intact. Power over your thoughts or reactions will place you in the right direction every time. Life has many facets and we do have choices to make because we only live once. Life is a gift that the fear monster is not yours to deal with anymore. It is someone else's problem now. You'll have the challenge of making good things happen in your life and surrounding yourself with great and good people. Smile, alas, go shopping to reward yourself with your new friend who goes by the name of "you in power." Today is your day for utter enjoyment of victory moreover courage yours to cherish for a lifetime.

# Dare 2 Forgive

*Zzzz---am I sleep…?*

Madness. Pissed off. Frustration. Stupidity. Rudeness. Ignorance. You may need to part with these dozens because you've dealt with many or all of these characters. These traits again are not yours and someone close around you keep carrying this monkey clan with them. It's horrible but what can you do? You've tried to help but help is an ancient secret to them. Plus your work is useless. "Us"-eless. Now, you tell yourself this is no more. Not this time around. Blam! It happens again and you didn't even get a warning sign. It is a life altering moment that could last a short period or longer term what do you do? The first response is to get mad possibly and make a rash decision. Next, you probably call people who are familiar with the present issue that has re-appeared yet again and again.

Here comes the band and everyone is saying the same conclusion to give up because you have wasted enough of your time. They tell you stories of long past what they've done and go on and on when all of a sudden your mind clicks back and forward to your present dilemma. You think about what river you have to cross to travel out of the stormy one to get to calmer water. Choices… help me God you may think. You have more conversations with earthly voices (people) who give favor and support to your situation because someone has to think bigger than the other.

You've cannot postpone that rational decision of forgiveness because you don't know how many monkeys exist with the toxic person. Fortunately in forgiveness you have to realize the back history of a person's behavior pattern and is there room for improvement? Did you witness a lot of unhappiness more so than happiness? Do you witness agony? No. What is needed is a friend instead of a foe you know el crazy person has already done the harm and if he or she have already beaten him or herself mentally then no more salt is needed for the wound. Miracles can happen along with this is the time for support and build positivism for the person. But you must deposit belief because it is powerful to truly re-invest in them and more over belief in them self is the key. One step at a time is the answer and love. Belief can move mountains and hopefully this person will see how blessed they really are as for the monkeys well let's just say that they're back at the zoo for once and for all. Forgiveness is powerful than revenge or abrupt thinking. To forgive is to be forgiven.

# Pressing Forward

*Is that a wall or not…?*

A stance is made between you and your challenger of placing your stability first. It will be an endeavor that you will finally have to rip yourself out in a thoughtful way. You don't have to raise your voice or be rude to someone but your point at this time is only meant to bring closure to your situation of disappointment. It is like you can't sleep peacefully at night until one day you say enough is enough. You have tried to stop the pattern of discomfort coming from the other person to you only to be mocked and laughed at. But… say to yourself he who laughs do not get the last laugh. It's true. The mockery in your mind has ceased and this is the beginning of pressing forward.

It might hurt or disappoint you but your future is everything to you in leaving a toxic person or situation behind. Loneliness may happen but you can find superior ways to occupy your time. Don't feel the hurt of moving on because you are not bringing that bad luggage into your present. You can't help or change certain people or circumstances so weigh the loss and shake the dust from your feet and move to better ground. In time all wounds heal and the sun is out again in you; people will see a better person in you. Never forget when you move forward and whatever was negative comes back to you a more improved human exemplifying brightness instead of pessimism then your pressing forward was a blessing in disguise. Sometimes the road is unclear until after your storm passes for you to see how all thing works together for those who love our Higher Power.

# I Can Do Anything Better or Like You

*You are in my mind...*

Some people are true innovators which don't FLAUNT it because it is natural. You are a different seed of people who are self-confident in caring not only for yourself but for others. There is a type of person who enjoys your company but underneath the smile is competition. You can involve yourself in a friendly relationship thinking everything is OK and being blinded at the same time because the competitor sheepishly wants what you've got. Does this remind you of someone?

The competitor looks at your life choices like career wise, car, children, etc. while deep down inside want out of their stick in the mud life and into yours. You get false smiles and weak conversations on how well the competitor's life is and remember this only camouflage because the conversation is not sincere and is very cunning plus deceptive in nature. Behold if you pay close attention little by little the competitor is transforming and imitating you. If you observe more closely the competitor really wants to become you so watch out and beware. It is time now to distance yourself because the relationship is going nowhere fast you don't owe anyone anything. The point is you don't need a wannabe person with a bad vibe around you. Avoid places or activities where you know the competitor will be for any given length of time. If this means going to lunch earlier or later then do it. If the competitor is an extended family member then pick and choose times when you will be at gathering and avoidance is your partner now you can enjoy yourself.

Don't give all your attention to the person and leave when you get ready. Competitors really don't like themselves because if they did then they would be happy with themselves. The only person to compete with is yourself to craft better and work at it every day. This is a sense of accomplishment that no one gave to you and no one can take it from you. So keep up your high-quality work and think twice of people who smile your face and have amnesia at the same time.

# Damned If I Do
# Damned If I Don't

*Need to keep my big mouth shut...*

You have people in life who always like to blame others for their problems. But the fact is that you are a good person always trying to give the best answer to others for advice. In your mind you feel you are doing the right thing to help someone else but you give yourself to others and others cannot see what you gave them was the best of your ability. They cannot fathom inside your consciousness of the great being that you are. So why keep pounding your head against the wall time after time after time after time. There is no happy medium and giving your good sound advice to people that inside of them don't have the capacity to discern what is going on or what is right and what is wrong with any circumstance.

So the best advice to give is to listen to your first mind because your first mind is the best mind. This is called first thought.

You will encounter people that are really miserable inside and the only way that they can make themselves feel better is by being mean while giving misery. Misery can be a demon of someone's past relationship with a mother, father, bad memory, or situation that cannot mentally or physically heal and grows into the abnormal minded person. An old saying says misery loves company and with this issue and someone else's life you have to realize when misery emerges and lunges at you with an attack. You feel yourself say something that really makes sense then you feel being blamed when you don't say something to a negative person.

The momentum you feel now is you are damned if you do say something or do something and you are damned if you don't with this person. In your mind and heart you know that when you done your deed it was in pure and perfect in context for the situation at hand because you treat people as you would treat self. But take a deep breath, breathe out, smile, and think to yourself… I can handle this because I have the solution for me and only me. Thus the only focus in this lifetime is to keep myself happy I cannot look to others to make me feel happy. Now the ball is rolling because you can make this bad situation turned positive and the key to the success is to remove yourself from this type of situation with this specific type of person.

You have allowed yourself over and over again to get caught in the "I'll be damned" trick bag. The best solution is not to give an opinion or advice to this type of person while letting them make their own decisions because by doing this that you have done flawlessly for yourself. Now, you have the control back in your hands for yourself because you no longer will get accused or blamed from that type of person who cannot see any fault in what they do. Time will come again when the blamer will talk to you but the best reaction is not to allow yourself to get involved in an any opinion or advice with this person. Let them handle what ever the problem, whatever the situation, whatever the circumstance is on their own. When you are asked a question pretend like you didn't hear it or say I don't know. Even if they make a mistake then it is their mistake put their misery back on them because they don't value your thoughtfulness or sound advice so you are really talking to a rock. This statement places the responsibility for the person to make a decision not you is the key.

Although you may have emotions like you don't want something to happen to this person and that is perfectly fine but you cannot keep allowing yourself to be blamed for someone else's fault. More than likely, they don't tell you the full truth concerning the specific details and after you have many irritating conversations that don't add up to anything with them because they speak in circles when you understood very well what was said to you in the initial conversation. You can see it is time to wakeup and stop your pattern of involvement. It is your pattern because you have allowed yourself time after time after time again to be victimized by the negative person once again. The fact remains that this person is never going to try to believe a good decision was made by you. The person goes through a spiral never seeing the middle hole which to make an exit for positivism and to let go the old ugly ways which hailing rain that keeps you in bad relationships or relations that you have no control over including the person either.

In life we have to take time to breathe because this is part of our exclusive existence. We have to take time to examine ourselves and the relationships that we share with others to see if the relationship is caring respectful, sharing, or is it filled with negativity and chaos and is the negativity and chaos always coming from the same person? We must know that this is why life is such a true gift that God has given each one of us to use. It's as a blessing to share with others who walk the earth knowing this best kept secret that is alive and well. Yet some people have dark hearts and cannot exhibit a peaceful persona or spirit and live for misfortune and bad relationships that never reach full capacity. So in turn, you have bent over backwards going well beyond your call of duty and had patience more than Job yet still there has not been a steady growth pattern for you to sustain your internal environment within your own inner being who has been abused and bruised in ways.

You must take time to assess the situation at hand to consciously excel privately to be quiet and brutally honest about the whole relationship between you and the negative person. Time has come for you to make a move. You have to make a final decision to rescue yourself and to keep you happy. You can only do this by taking the plunge to limit your conversation with this person; two things can happen either you can dissolve the relationship or you can keep the relationship and the conversations brief. Brief means hi and bye or see ya don't want to be ya.

It can only be simple but as just mentioned because either you're going to sink or swim and it is time to swim.

Finding the strength that you have in yourself can be overwhelming sometimes just remember this trend is always residing in side of you and all you have to do is take the consorted effort and time to release it and get yourself back on track. You only have one life to live. This statement can be said over and over again until it's resonates in your brain to focus on and live by because a happy person can live a long life.

# My Work Is Done

*How I Got Over --- I Look Back And Wonder...*

At some point in your life you've had a person project and this project required a lot of your mental and emotional powers. A person project consists of sacrificing oneself because you saw a dire need in another person's misfortunate life. Now let's examine misfortune. Misfortune has many faces which are attributed to many childhood psychological problems in which an adult has not confronted to alleviate themselves from their demons. The demons act as obstacles and forces that are self-inducing and self-distracting in every nature of the person who can't seem to rid themselves of being self destructive by staying in trouble, being absolutely negative, or not using discernment to ever grow and mature as an adult.

You see the people project as an opportunity to do well and make a difference in someone's life. It takes a special person of favorable character to embark on such a dismal at times mission to complete the person project. Your impulse is to help someone because somewhere you have a direct connection with this person and in some form you might feel like it's your obligation to help them to get back on the right track to do well for themselves and others. One of the main reasons that you accept this mission is because you probably see potential in this person when others see nothing so you hone your attention on what could be a positive change in direction for that person. At some point you may even feel like you're the mother or father to this person which is a natural emotion to hold in your psyche because somewhere down the line the person has missed love, time, and discipline from parental guidance.

In your mission you have now taken on being a parent, counselor, and disciplinarian for the human being. At times you can see and welcome the positive changes within the person. On the contrary, you get rebellion from the creature because any wrongs within them self is not seen. This is exactly where the problem starts because now the demons have blocked the rational and common sense thinking of that person; you see before your eyes manifesting a totally different person other than the calm, nice, and happy person who you decided to help in the first place. In your mind, emotionally you feel disappointed while thinking this being is an adult who acts like a child because they cannot discern their thoughts; you know right from wrong in doing good and bad. What makes a relationship happy or what makes a relationship sad. We can also take this issue in further because some people are reared by their mom and dad but choose to be selfish and live by their own destructive ways. The sad irony is that this person knows exactly what he or she is doing. The individual is not retarded and do have plenty of good sense but chooses to go down the rough road of life not caring about other people who've surrounded the person.

There comes a time when you hear a consensus from other people who are connected to this one person and they all say the same negative traits about this individual in which you already know and encountered. Profoundly this has to be a wake up call because in life when everybody says the same thing about one person then it has got to be true especially when everyone doesn't know each other. It is a crying shame that the creature is so discombobulated and thinks everything is simply marvelous, there is nothing wrong, and like chaos then your only alternative is to retreat. Give up because you are fighting a losing battle. You hate to give up on this person but you have to shake the dust from your feet and keep moving because their issues are more than you can handle. This may be a hard task to encounter for yourself since you have invested so much time in and with the individual and somewhere deep inside yourself you still believe there is opportunity for change and advancement to be stable. But your reality check is to know that unfortunately the work is done; you have to realize that you've come to the mountaintop of possible methods to help someone to make life a better space and time. It will not work out as you have desired. Point blank, it just won't work. You have come to the end of your road---it's a wrap.

Your next step is to heal. You are emotional because you've invested so much of yourself into this person and mentally in addition to somewhat physical you are drained. Face it…you have been defeated. It will be hard to let go and walk away, but you have to conjure the strength to let it happen or you're going to crash and burn yourself by remaining in a bad situation. Now do whatever it takes for yourself to get back on track. The goal is to go anywhere you'd like to and visit or talk with people you enjoy being around to begin the healing process. You only have one life that God has given you to enjoy and be fruitful. It's OK to throw in the towel and walk out a winner because you and no one else but you… took on the responsibility to try and help another to self-improve. So there is no discussion whatsoever to demean you for what you tried to accomplish. There are not a lot of people out in the world that would take on the role of sacrifice that you done. Hats off to you and go do something good for yourself this day forward to enjoy life… the rest of your life. All things must come to an end and the end is where something far greater begins.

## ABOUT THE AUTHOR

Pattie Thomas has worked in the entertainment industry for more than fourteen years in theatre, radio, film, and television. She helped the movement of arts and culture in Chicago by using her expertise, love for the arts, and mentoring individuals. After her first degree in Speech and Broadcasting, she worked at CBS WBBM Radio as an assistant producer. Pattie holds a master's degree in Media & Business Management as well. She currently lives in Illinois with her two children and granddaughter.

You are invited to post comments at pattiethomas7@yahoo.com.

Made in the USA
Lexington, KY
13 May 2010